THE NATURE OF CAREGIVING

Photographs and Words to Inspire Self-Care

By Rebecca S. Hauder, RN, M.Ed.

Published by Resources for Grief™
Boise, ID 83702
www.resourcesforgrief.com

THE NATURE OF CAREGIVING

Photos and Text: Rebecca S. Hauder, RN, M.Ed.

For information, contact Resources for Grief: info@resourcesforgrief.com, or visit www.resourcesforgrief.com

ISBN 13: 978-1-5193-5232-3
Printed in the United States of America

March 2020

To the dedicated and compassionate caregivers
who give of their time, energy and talents
to care for patients or loved ones
too ill or frail to care for themselves.

Crystal –
I hope these words and pictures
help you nurture yourself as
you care for so many, at work and
at home. Thank you for all you
do and all you are.
Love,
Holly

Contents

Introduction–vii

Consider Self-Care a Part-Time Job–3

Cultivate Gratitude–5

Own Your Feelings–7

Acknowledge the Sacred–9

Ask for Help–11

Accept Your Vulnerabilities–13

Strive for Balance–15

Breathe Slowly–17

Keep Perspective–19

Count to 10 When Triggered–21

Memorize a Prayer or Mantra–23

Leave Your Shoes at the Door–25

Recognize Your Limits–27

Establish Boundaries–29

Eat Wisely–31

Maintain Hope–33

Seek Outlets for Difficult Emotions–35

Discover the Power of Two Questions–37

Eliminate the Non-Essentials–39
Adapt to Changing Circumstances–41
Learn to Compartmentalize–43
Exercise–45
Monitor Your Attitude–47
Laugh Often–49
Lean Not on Your Own Understanding–51
Nurture Your Close Relationships–53
Live with Authenticity–55
Stay Hydrated–57
Be Where You Are–59
Grieve the Losses–61
Take Your N Vitamin–63
Respond Creatively to Mistreatment–65
Slow Down, Be Present–67
Get Your Sleep–69
Keep a Journal–71
Choose to Forgive–73
Make Time for Leisure–75
Practice Equanimity–77
Seek Support–79
Let Go–81

Introduction

The nurses who hovered over me in my hospital bed when I was a very ill twelve-year-old exuded kindness, compassion, and a desire to ease my pain and fears. I left Bethel Deaconess two weeks later pretty certain I wanted to be a nurse. That dream eventually was realized, thanks to the support and encouragement of my family who believed service to others was key to making their Mennonite Christian faith real. Nearly twenty years later, after a fulfilling nursing career in a variety of settings, including hospitals, home health, hospice, and a clinic in the slums of Kingston, Jamaica, my desire to care for others remains, though my focus has now shifted to mental health.

The motivation and inspiration for most professionally trained caregivers, including myself, is to help alleviate the pain of others in some way. Often arising out of a personal experience with suffering, this is their passion and calling. Yet, I would be remiss not to mention that there are countless others providing day-to-day caregiving out of a sense of duty or necessity. In this role, they may find profound significance and meaning, or they may acknowledge that caregiving is primarily an exercise of patience and endurance.

Whether we as caregivers are trained or untrained, paid or unpaid, professional or lay, our role does have an underbelly—that is, a side not often seen by others. Most folks, in fact, see us as living saints!

Nonetheless, there's an underbelly to this work that needs attention! It's the part of us that keeps plugging away, even when the workload is too heavy, the emotional toll from watching someone suffer too great, the sense of isolation too burdensome (particularly for family caregivers), and the lack of time for recreation, recuperation, family and friends too costly. Some days, concerns unrelated to caregiving compound the strain and stress factor even further.

Yes, providing care to others is demanding work. And, if we wish to stay effective and fulfilled for the long haul, we must find ways to minimize the hazard—the drive that keeps us giving and giving while ignoring the warning signs that our life is sorely out of balance. As Ralph Waldo Emerson, famous lecturer and poet, once said, "No person can sincerely try to help another without helping themselves." In a similar vein, he said, "If you would lift me up, you must be on higher ground." In other words, we can't be at our best as caregivers if we haven't first provided for our own needs—if we aren't any healthier than the one we're caring for. Otherwise, we increase our chances of illness, accidents, relationship difficulties, emotional problems, exhaustion, irritability, and burnout. It's humanly impossible to properly help and support another without also attending to our own wellbeing.

If you're saying, "Yes, I agree, but I don't have the time, motivation, know-how, energy, or resources," then these pages are for you. The brief self-care tips contained in this book (And I mean brief, because I know you don't have a lot of time!) are designed to inspire, encourage, educate, and support.

Because I believe in a life of balance and equilibrium, there are chapters encouraging care of the body, mind, emotions, spirit, and relationships. Also, you'll see chapters that provide specific caregiving strategies. I've grouped these topics together in the Topical Index in the back of the book, but as you can see from the Table of Contents, these topics are intermixed so that you'll get a balanced set of tips if you read the book from beginning to end.

Quoting Christian monk and mystic, Thomas Merton, "Happiness is not a matter of intensity but of balance and order and rhythm and harmony." While you may never achieve the balance and order you hope for, particularly as you care for others, your striving will put you on the journey toward a happier, healthier, and more effective you.

~ *Rebecca S. Hauder*

Photographs and Words to Inspire Self-Care

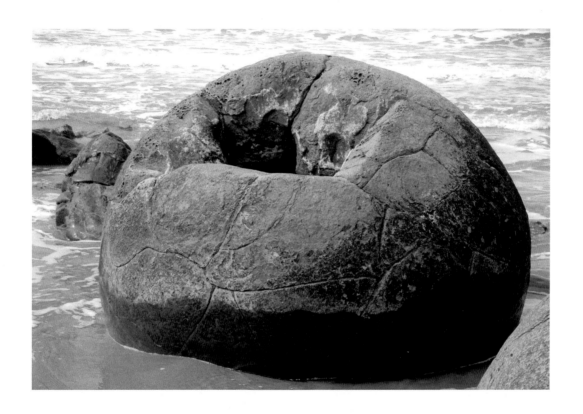

"Self-care is not selfish.
You cannot serve from an empty vessel."   ~ Eleanor Brownn

Consider Self-Care a Part-Time Job

It's winter as I write this, and the weather has been downright depressing. Six weeks of little to no sunshine has had a cumulative effect on my spirit. Exercise has been a chore, and I've had little motivation to lose the extra pounds I gained over the holidays.

Into this stupor of self-neglect, I attended a noon seminar on the topic of healthy aging. There, I learned that the same tactics known to reduce the risk of cancer and other diseases—a healthy diet, adequate sleep, regular exercise, spiritual practices, and fostering friendships—are also the keys to healthy aging. What else is new? I thought. But when, near the conclusion of the presentation, the speaker suggested we consider self-care a part-time job, it struck a chord! I'm conscientious and do my best when fulfilling a job, whether or not I'm in the mood. I could look at exercise and the cultivation of other healthy habits the same way!

I realize another job is hardly what you, a hardworking caregiver, want or think you need, but nonetheless, self-care must be given part-time job status! The person receiving your care is dependent upon you staying mentally and physically healthy, and the practices that promote this state of well-being take time! As a reminder to yourself, place a note in a prominent place that reads, "Self-care is my new part-time job!"

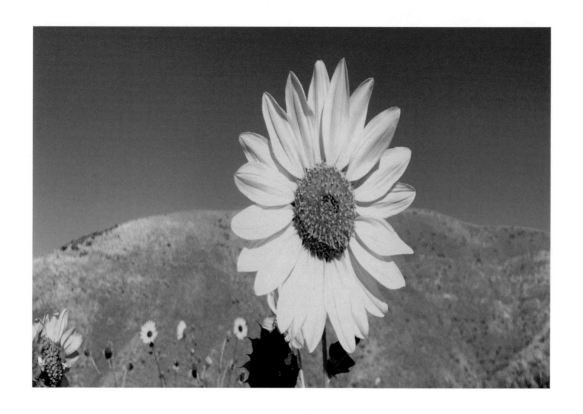

"If the only prayer you said in your whole life was 'thank you,' that would suffice."   ~ Meister Eckhart

Cultivate Gratitude

Recently I granted an interview to a counseling student to help her fulfill a class assignment. While I was not eager to spend one more hour of a sunny spring day in my office, the beautiful floral bouquet Keisha handed me as she walked in the door, a beaming smile on her face, demonstrated her regard for my time. Feeling appreciated, I gave her my undivided attention. Her gratitude benefited us both.

Noticing, then acknowledging, the things we appreciate in others, in ourselves, and in our day-to day living is a great antidote to unhappiness and depression! And study after study proves the physical health benefits as well, including an improved ability to fight off infection!

A powerful way to nurture a grateful heart is to write down five big or little joys at the end of each day. Your list might include a hot shower, a lunchtime walk, a meaningful encounter, a compliment received, or your own handling of a difficult situation. To demonstrate your gratefulness to others, particularly those who assist and support you, regularly acknowledge their positive qualities. And don't overlook the person(s) for whom you're giving care; they too need recognition, perhaps for their patience, humor, cooperation, positive attitude, or for what they have taught you.

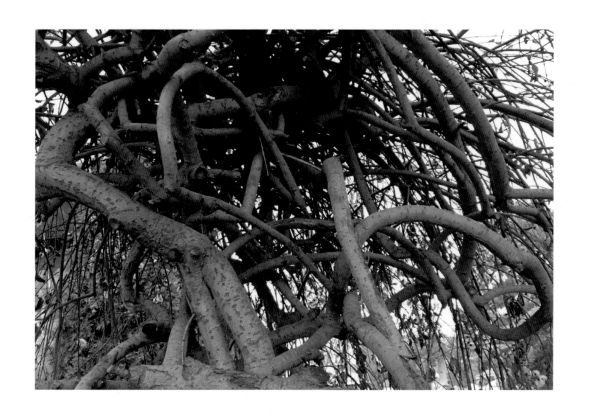

"What we resist persists."

~ C.G. Jung

Own Your Feelings

Alena and her fiancé invited her dad, who had stage four cancer, to live with them during his final days. After two weeks, both caregivers were worn thin, not because they begrudged the commitment, but because her father was so demanding and grouchy! Alena started feeling angry and resentful, and, at the same time, guilty for feeling angry.

Intense and conflicting emotions go hand-in-hand with caregiving; they are not right or wrong, good or bad. Our task is simply to acknowledge and accept whatever emotions we experience. Then we're less apt to expend precious energy fighting or denying their existence, often through overeating, overdrinking, overworking, or overspending. What emotions, listed below, have a familiar ring to you? Are there others you can list?

~ Anxiety and Fear: The future is unknown for me, and for the one receiving my care.
~ Helplessness: No matter how much I do, there is still so much I cannot do!
~ Anger: A sense of frustration and helplessness is often at the root of my anger.
~ Resentfulness: Time for myself is no more; neither is time with friends and family.
~ Guilt: I tell myself I'm not doing enough, or that I've been impatient.
~ Sadness: Watching a patient or loved one struggle or decline is tough!
~ Grief: Anticipating a death, I face my own mortality, and grieve prior losses.

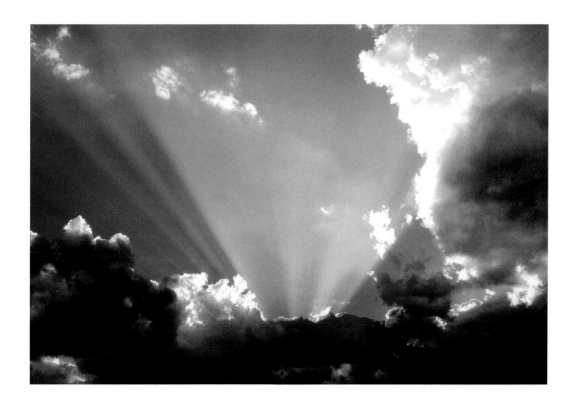

"As you engage in the simple acts of care, you may begin to witness signs that the Divine is in your midst."   ~ Rev. James E. Miller

Acknowledge the Sacred

With a degree of trepidation, I headed out of the hospice office parking lot to visit Joe. His edgy and prickly demeanor on my two previous visits made me cautious with my words. I tried to be attentive and respectful, but truth be told, I stayed as short a time as possible—just long enough to accomplish my nursing tasks—before making an exit.

Future visits to Joe fortunately softened my attitude, particularly as I saw glimpses of the fearful vulnerable person beneath the prickly facade. I considered how tough it would it be to have a life full of plans and expectations suddenly go awry because of an out-of-the-blue stage-four cancer diagnosis; then three months later to be receiving care from a complete stranger! Putting myself in his shoes helped me empathize and listen more intently to the feelings behind his words. He, in turn, became more open about his fear of losing control. A sacred space seemed to envelop both of us in those honest and profound exchanges.

Henri Nouwen, in *The Spirituality of Caregiving*, writes, "Caregiving carries within it an opportunity for inner healing, liberation, and transformation for the one being cared for and for the one who cares." Can you identify a time when you experienced a transformative and sacred moment as you've provided care to another?

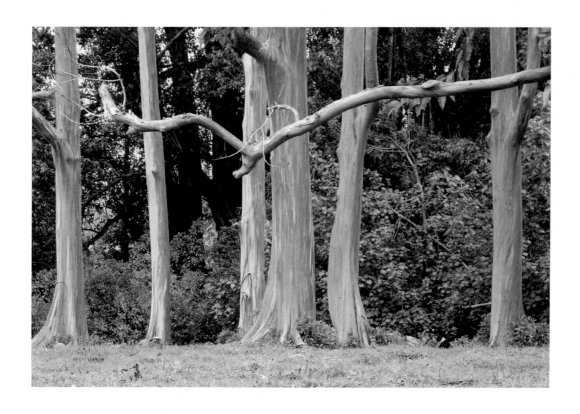

"It's not the load that breaks you down;
it's the way you carry it."   ~ Lena Horne

Ask for Help

A fellow parishioner called recently to ask if I would bring a meal to him and his wife. Knowing his wife was suffering the effects of chemotherapy had prompted me to make offers previously, but he had always declined help, until the day he courageously reached out. I was pleased he called, as preparing a meal was a tangible way to assist.

Asking for and accepting help is difficult! Who likes to be dependent on others, especially if there's a chance they won't do things our way or according to our standards and timetable? But thinking we can or must do it all ourselves is a counterproductive trap, one that most of us have fallen victim to at one time or another. The reality is, we will achieve more than we ever could on our own by enlisting the help of others! And those we call on are likely to feel honored we asked. Nonetheless, I think it's important to keep in mind some common-sense rules of etiquette before soliciting another's assistance:

~ Pinpoint what needs to be done and approximately how much time it will take.
~ Try not to pile on other tasks when someone comes to assist.
~ Say thank-you. People are more apt to help again if they feel appreciated.
~ Finally, congratulate yourself for asking!

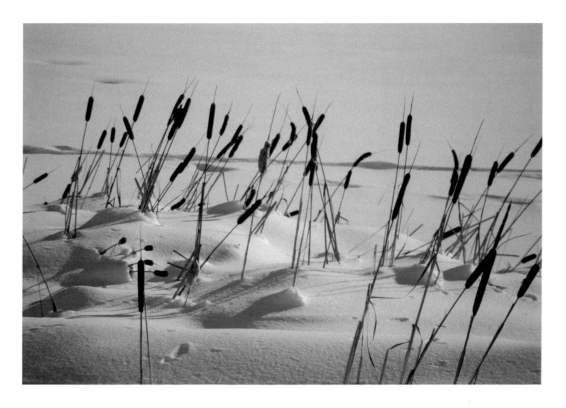

"When we were children, we used to think that when we were grown-up we would no longer be vulnerable. But to grow up is to accept vulnerability...To be alive is to be vulnerable."

~ Madeleine L'Engle

Accept Your Vulnerabilities

My Grandson loves superhero action figures. These bigger-than-life characters were of no particular interest to me until Luke's enthusiasm attracted my curiosity. I've discovered that most superheroes have vulnerabilities, in spite of their superhuman powers. Kryptonite, for instance, poses as a threat to Superman.

Caregivers, particularly those who serve the dying, are often viewed as superheroes. "You are amazing," or, "I could never do what you do," are common responses. Yet, in spite of the important and gratifying nature of their work, caregivers aren't immune from vulnerabilities, including stress responses and compassion fatigue. Ignoring those symptoms is common, however, particularly since their attention is drawn to those with greater needs. Plus, helpers often have difficulty admitting weakness and vulnerability.

Are you currently noticing any "threats" to your role as caregiver? These threats, or vulnerabilities, may include feeling consistently overwhelmed, worn out, apathetic, and unhappy. A preoccupation with the one(s) you're caring for, poor sleep, difficulty concentrating, and chronic physical problems are common caregiver vulnerabilities as well. If and when you first notice these threatening signs, take action! Identify and initiate some self-care practices that can start to restore you—mind, body, and spirit.

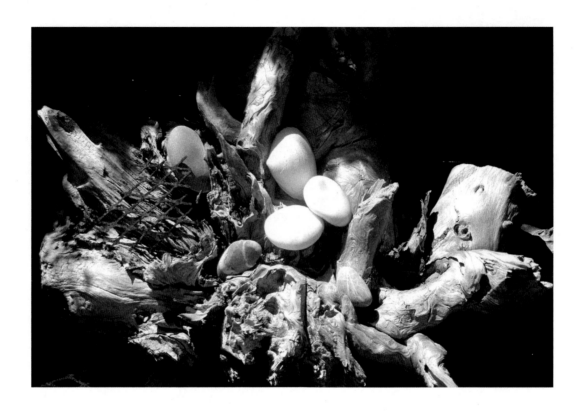

"Happiness is not a matter of intensity, but of balance and order and rhythm and harmony."   ~ Thomas Merton

Strive for Balance

In yoga class, the one-legged balancing poses are often the most challenging for me. Along with finding my center of gravity, I am required to stay alert and focused while also remembering to breathe. Some days, unsteadiness makes this "tree pose" nearly impossible. Other times, when muscles, bones, thoughts, and emotions are all in alignment, I maintain the pose with relative ease.

Balancing the daily routines and rituals of life is much like a yoga practice. A sense of harmony prevails when I stay focused on priorities: eating regular nutritious meals, getting some exercise, going to religious services, sleeping eight hours at night, and spending time with friends and family. But I feel "off" when a number of days go by without the activities that keep me emotionally and physically stable, as tends to be the reality when I'm in caregiver mode. Then, others' needs take front and center as mine fade to the background. For short periods, I manage quite well with a disrupted schedule and lack of balance. However, over the longer haul, I notice that irritability, anger, depression, and physical maladies begin to surface.

What symptoms are reminders that your life is off-kilter? What rituals or practices bring back a sense of balance and stability? How do you incorporate these when caregiving?

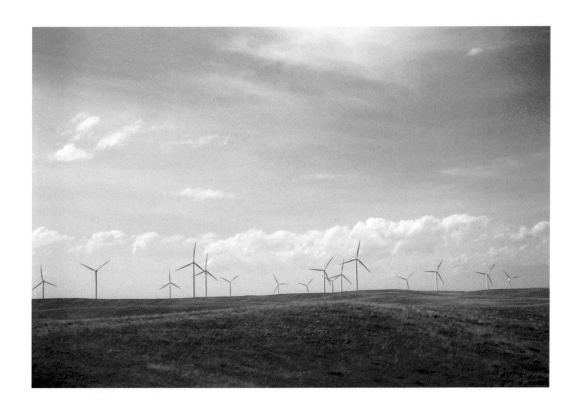

"Feelings come and go like clouds in a windy sky.
Conscious breathing is my anchor."   ~ Thich Nhat Hanh

Breathe Slowly

Eva arrived in my counseling office last week, anxious and upset about a near accident she had driving to our appointment. After debriefing with her about the incident, I coached her in a simple breathing technique to help her relax. Here were my instructions:

1. Sit in a comfortable position in a chair or on the floor. Close your eyes.
2. Count to four as you breathe in slowly through your nose, pausing briefly at the end of your inhale.
3. Count to six as you breathe out slowly through your nose.
4. Breathe in and out slowly for several minutes, remembering to make your exhalations a little longer than your inhalations.

During tense times, I often practice this method of breathing. It's a quick and effective way to quiet my body and mind. With this type of breathing, the vagus nerve—connecting my diaphragm and brainstem—signals my brain to calm down and relax. The brain in turn sends this message to my body, causing a drop in my heart rate and blood pressure, a reduction in stress hormones, and an increase in energy. Now, try it for yourself, at least once a day, and notice the difference in how you feel!

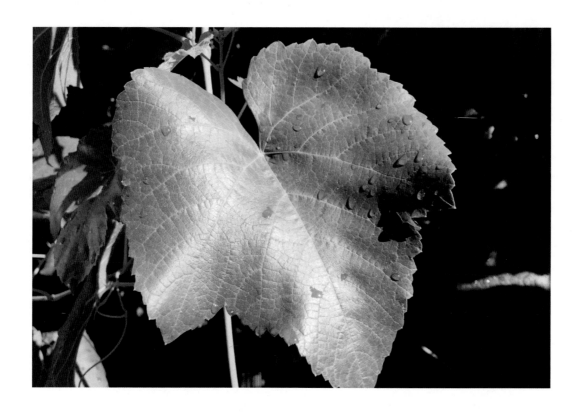

"The plant grows in the mist and under clouds as truly as under sunshine."   ~ William Ellery Channing

Keep Perspective

Worried and frazzled best describes the emotional state of my friend, Jenny, in our half-hour phone conversation. Both her mom and her daughter were experiencing serious health crises, and Jenny was providing childcare as well as financial and emotional support during this uncertain time. A huge disappointment was her needing to cancel a long-awaited trip to Europe, and Jenny wondered aloud whether she'd ever have this opportunity again.

Perhaps you can relate to Jenny's situation, feeling cheated because you too have had to put plans on hold due to current caregiving responsibilities. In fact, you might assume your "on hold" status will go on forever—that you'll never have a life again! "Overgeneralization" is a label for this kind of thinking. It assumes your current situation is part of a never-ending pattern of defeat. And, because it fosters a sense of helplessness and hopelessness, it's an unhealthy perspective to maintain.

When you find yourself overgeneralizing, try looking at your situation from a different perspective. Even though your current plans, goals, and ambitions have been altered, they're not necessarily lost. Rather, your hopes for the future could unknowingly be evolving into something new and different, possibly even better.

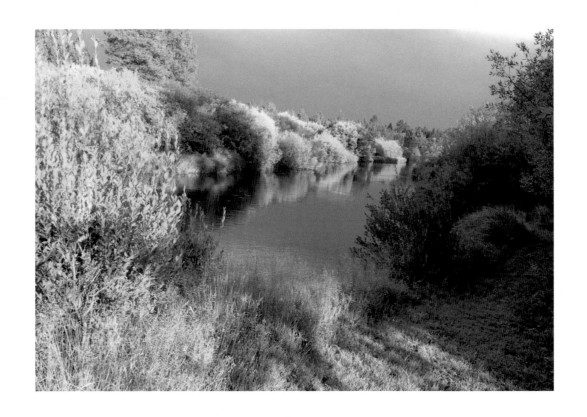

"Calmness is the cradle of power."   ~ J.G. Holland

Count to 10 When Triggered

Sabra, a caregiver for her elderly parents, told me how she blew up at her older sister last week when her sister called to offer unsolicited advice about their parents' care. The advice-giving had happened one too many times and Sabra could no longer contain herself. Now the relationship between them was cool and tense.

We all experience situations that trigger intense emotions like anger, rage, and panic! Maybe it's a coworker not doing their fair share, a child's snide remark, or a patient's unreasonable demands. Whatever the cause of our upset, the stress hormone, adrenalin, is activated, and we readily feel its effects, including a rapid pulse and quickened breathing! Our ability to think clearly is also diminished, and we're apt to respond irrationally with a roll of the eyes, an exasperated sigh, or a shout. These reactions cause us embarrassment and sometimes create long-lasting hostilities.

Next time you get triggered, take a step back. Become aware of your emotions and bodily responses. Then, self-soothe by breathing slowly and deeply, or count to 10 as you learned to do as a child. Finally, when you have cooled down, calmly address, with the person who upset you, the issue at hand. Remember that calmness is more likely to bring respect and power than a hotheaded response.

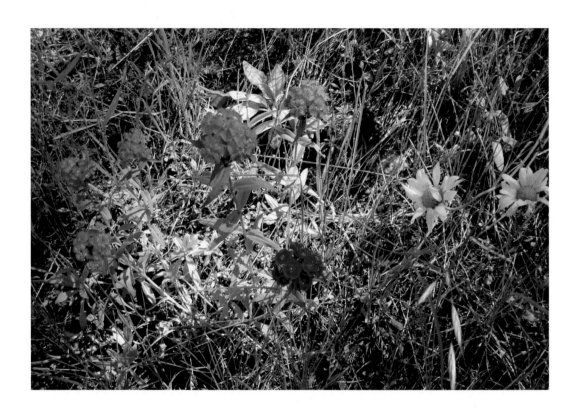

"May peace and love fill my heart, beauty fill my world,
contentment and joy fill my day."   ~ Anonymous

Memorize a Prayer or Mantra

Last week, the chorus of a song played repeatedly in my mind long after hearing it on the radio. Frequently I found myself humming or singing the catchy tune, until it faded away—finally! Neuroscientists call this phenomenon "earworms."

Prayers and mantras—short phrases repeated over and over—can be a kind of "earworm." Recited anywhere, anytime, they help redirect our thoughts. When utilized upon awakening, a prayer or mantra jump-starts our day with a sense of appreciation and optimism. The Book of Psalms has many passages that can be used for this purpose. For example: "This is the day that the Lord has made; let us rejoice and be glad in it" (Psalm 118:24). The quote on the adjacent page is another meaningful prayer for the start of a day. Repetitive prayers are also useful under stress. This is one I find helpful: "May I dwell in my heart; May I be free from suffering; May I be healed; May I be at peace." I vary the words to fit the situation, and, when concerned for another, I use "he, "she," or "they" in place of "I."

A two-week experiment: Memorize a repetitious prayer, song, poem, verse, or mantra. Repeat it every morning and during challenging or stressful times throughout the day. Notice if or how it changes your attitude and the way you relate to others.

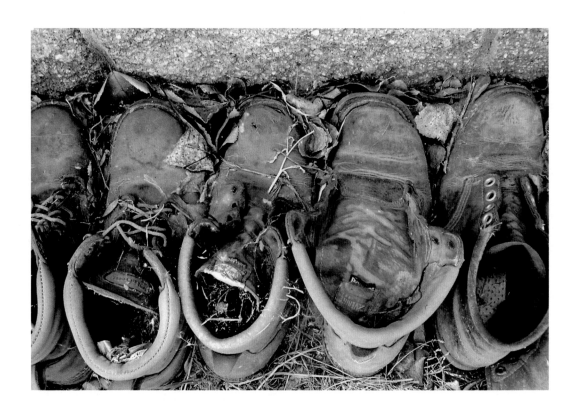

"Leave your worries and your shoes at the door."

~Anonymous

Leave Your Shoes at the Door

We have friends in Seattle who remind us, when we visit, to leave our shoes at the door. They don't like dust and dirt from the outside brought inside. I admire their commitment to this practice, even though it's not one I've consistently implemented in our home.

Leaving shoes at the door is an appropriate metaphor for putting my caregiving concerns aside when I'm off-duty or taking a break. When precious time away is spent ruminating on what I should have said or done, worrying about all I have to do, or responding to texts, calls, or emails related to work, I pollute my off-time and pass up the opportunity for needed rest and renewal.

I've developed some rituals over the years to help me "leave my shoes at the door" when entering my world apart from caregiving. Those have included writing a to-do list before leaving my job so it doesn't occupy off-duty mind space; washing my hands, and/or donning a fresh change of clothes when entering my non-work environment; and, taking a few deep breaths as I walk away from my helper role—breathing in gratefulness for the positive aspects of my day and breathing out any negativity.

What rituals help you step away from your role as caregiver when you're off-duty?

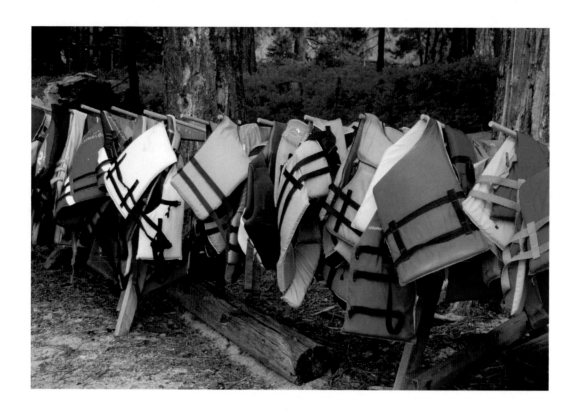

"Pride does not suffice as a flotation device
if your ship is sinking in flames."   ~ Jim Deters

Recognize Your Limits

During my tenure as a hospice nurse, a close friend died of AIDS. After her death, and for the next several months, I found myself overcome with intense emotions when caring for patients with AIDS. Not wanting to appear weak, I tried to keep my chin up and go on performing my duties, but it became increasingly difficult. Quitting my job began to look like the best alternative, as I felt too embarrassed to tell anyone about my situation. After all, the other team members seemed so strong and unflappable.

As it turned out, I didn't quit my job, but swallowed my hospice nurse pride long enough to let my supervisor know about my emotional state. Without hesitation, she encouraged me to continue working, but suggested I not be assigned to patients with AIDS for several months until I experienced some emotional healing.

Given a needed break, I was finally able to resume my full caregiving responsibilities, but I learned some important lessons in the process that have stayed with me to this day: First, there are limits to what I can do. Second, denying my limits is foolish and irrational. Third, admitting my limits is not a weakness, but instead promotes self-respect, integrity, and emotional health.

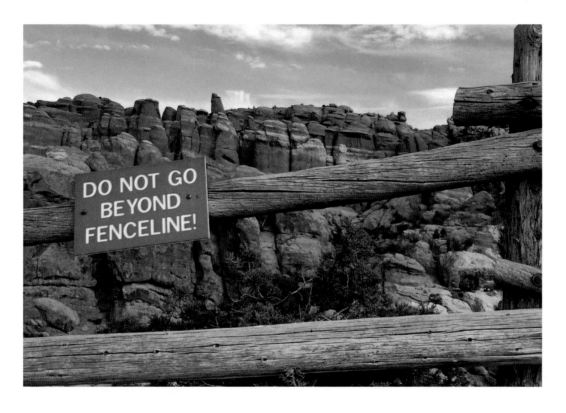

"Daring to set boundaries is about having the courage to love
ourselves, even when we risk disappointing others."

~ Brene Brown

Establish Boundaries

Scenario #1: Janet's mother had Alzheimer's and was eventually placed in a memory care facility. Janet, feeling guilty she could no longer keep her mother at home, visited everyday after work, often eating dinner with her. Janet's husband complained of feeling slighted, to no avail. Their marriage grew strained and finally dissolved.

Scenario #2: Maria, a home care bath aide, visited patient Bob outside of regular work hours, sometimes bringing him her homemade goodies. When Maria went out of town for a week, and another bath aide showed up at the house, Bob refused her assistance. "I'll wait until Maria returns," he said.

A tendency we caregivers have is to give too much—more than what is necessary—because we want to please; plus, having another depend on us can feed our ego. But, over-caring comes at a big cost! Family and friends are often neglected, personal needs get overlooked, and an unhealthy dependency develops by the one(s) receiving our care. And so, the need for boundaries! Boundaries give us permission to say "no" when we are tired or in need of a break, and boundaries protect all parties from emotional harm. As Robert Frost wrote in his poem, *Mending Wall*: "Good fences make good neighbors." And I say, "Good fences also make good caregivers!"

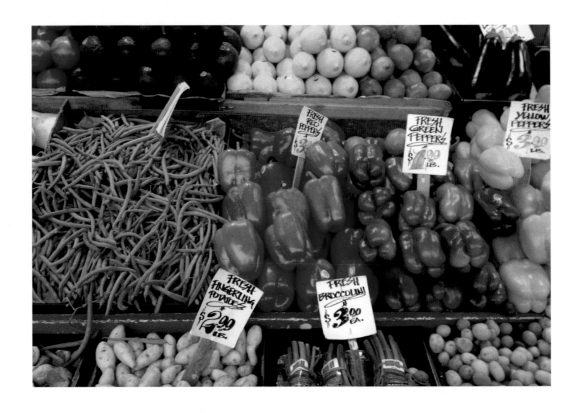

"Those who have no time for healthy eating will sooner or later have to find time for illness."   ~Edward Stanley

Eat Wisely

When taking care of my young grandchildren for all or part of a day, I often ignore my bodily cues for hunger and thirst. I make my little darlings breakfast, lunch, and snacks in between, but neglect to do the same for myself. Eventually, I feel the twinges of low blood sugar and grab whatever's in sight—animal cookies, potato chips, or leftover crusts of grilled cheese sandwiches.

When hurried and stressed, our tendency is to eat fast and impulsively, with little thought about a food item's nutritional value or what it's doing to our bodies. But, at least the hunger pangs and emotional distress are temporarily quelled. High carb "junk food" fills us up fast, but when the blood sugar crashes a while later, we feel fatigued, irritable, and have trouble focusing. Plus, we're apt to put on some unneeded pounds.

What to do? First, be aware of everything you put in your mouth. Second, keep a stash of healthy high-protein snacks on hand—nuts, pumpkin seeds, celery or apple slices with peanut butter, cheese sticks, hard-boiled eggs, cut-up veggies with hummus. These supply quick energy to the body and help maintain a stable blood sugar level. Lastly, plan meals and snacks in advance, before heading to the grocery store. Then you're less apt to stop for fast-food, which is often high in calories and low on nutrients.

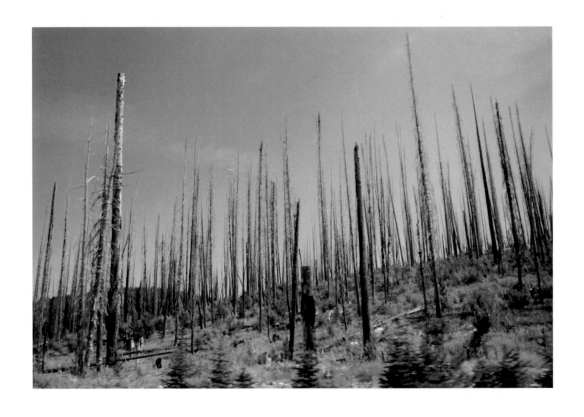

"To live without hope is to cease to live."   ~ Fyodor Dostoevsky

Maintain Hope

Recently I rode my bicycle through an area of Central Idaho that had burned in a 1994 forest fire. After twenty years, blackened tree trunks still stand like matchsticks against the blue-sky backdrop. At a glance, the landscape appears sparse, barren, and lifeless.

I stopped along the road to capture a photo of the desolation, and noticed the varieties of vegetation that had taken root in the rich soil containing ash and decayed wood. An informational sign titled "New Wildlife Habitat" explained that deer, elk, coyote, black bear, and ground-foraging birds favor the reduced forest cover and rich plant life that has emerged. Small animals and insects have benefited as well. Life has returned to a forest once in ruins!

As caregivers, we're confronted with a variety of tragedies and losses that can be devastating for us and for those who receive our care. The future can look bleak and overwhelming for what seems like a very long time. The metaphor of a forest fire is a reminder that even though life seems pretty depressing at times, it's not likely to stay that way. Over time—sometimes at a snail's pace—new life emerges out of the ash and stubble. While that "new life" will look different for each person and situation, we must remember that hope does lie beyond despair, even in life's most trying times.

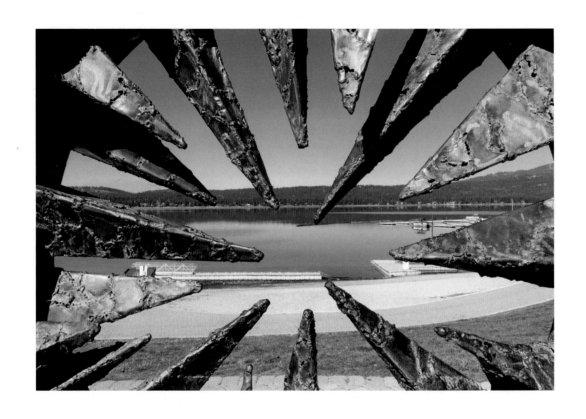

"We must embrace pain and burn it as fuel for our journey."
~ Kenji Miyazawa

Seek Outlets for Difficult Emotions

When I'm anxious, my hands get cold and clammy. When I feel unprepared or insecure prior to giving a presentation, I get "butterflies" in my stomach. And when I get angry, my jaw tightens. These, and a myriad of other physical sensations, offer the first clues of intense and difficult emotions.

But, why is paying attention to these bodily cues so important? Paying attention brings emotions to the forefront where I can work with them. When suppressed, these emotions cause wear and tear on my body and cause me to turn to unhealthy behaviors in an effort to cope. Therefore, I have a first-aid plan for handling difficult emotions. I'll share it here in hopes it will benefit you as well:

~ **Accept** whatever you're feeling. Emotions are not right or wrong, good or bad.

~ **Identify** your feelings; give them a name. Notice the cues in your body.

~ **Do** something with your feelings; they need a safe outlet in a time, place, and manner of your choosing: Cry. Go for a walk. Talk to someone who will listen without judging. Depict your feelings with crayons or paint. Write a letter you don't send expressing the anger you feel. Putting your words on paper is not dishonoring of anyone; rather, it helps you gain freedom and release!

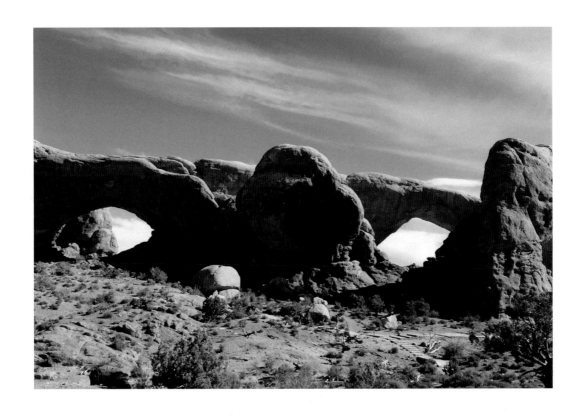

"People generally see what they look for, and hear
what they listen for. . ."   ~ Harper Lee

Discover the Power of Two Questions

As caregiver to his wife with advanced M.S., my client felt isolated, exhausted, and emotionally drained. Furthermore, the relentless demands of caregiving made it difficult for him to stand back, reflect, and gain perspective on the situation. He needed a caregiver for himself! I suggested he try a daily Examen practice, hoping to encourage daily self-awareness and counter his difficult and negative emotions.

Examen is a two-question process taking just five minutes, but with many longer-lasting benefits. Credited to St. Ignatius, Examen is a way to reflect on the positive and negative aspects of each day. It requires setting aside a short period of time in a quiet comfortable spot—ideally at the end of the day. Here are the simple directions:

1. Take several deep breaths to help quiet your body and mind.
2. Ask yourself: For what moment today am I most grateful? Breathe in gratitude as you remember that moment.
3. Ask yourself: For what moment today am I the least grateful? Consider what made it so difficult—without passing judgment on yourself or others.
4. Give thanks to God, or a higher power, for all you experienced this day.
5. If you have time, jot down your responses.

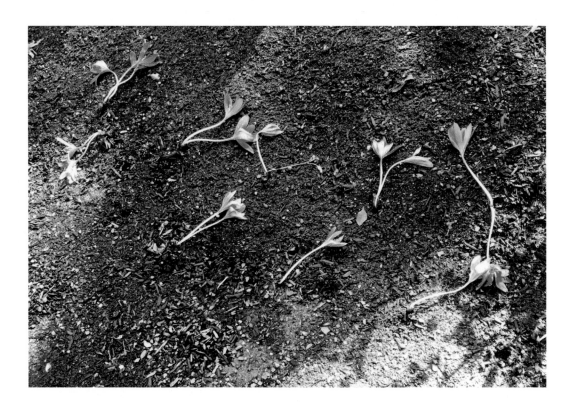

"Besides the noble art of getting things done, there is the noble art of leaving things undone. The wisdom of life consists in the elimination of non-essentials."   ~ Lin Yutang

Eliminate the Non-Essentials

I find it hard to relax when there are dishes in the sink, cluttered counters, or a dirty kitchen floor. However, when my grandchildren come to visit, I prioritize time with them over everyday household tasks. Keeping them occupied, happy, and safe is my goal. The dishes, floors, and counter can wait; they are non-essentials.

Focusing on the essentials, leaving some things undone, is crucial for all caregivers. Otherwise, the numerous duties and responsibilities can be overwhelming! Giving medications, running errands, fixing meals, assisting with baths, paying bills, handling insurance claims, providing emotional support, making decisions, coordinating care with health care professionals, and communicating with family members are some of the most common of tasks. In addition, caregivers usually have a myriad of other responsibilities that have nothing to do with caregiving!

If you, a caregiver, are feeling overwhelmed with your lengthy to-do list, cross off as many of the would-be-nice-but-not-essential items as you possibly can! For instance, leave the furniture undusted; change sheets on the beds less often; allow some weeds in the flowerbeds; and refrain from making that obligatory, but unnecessary, phone call. Small tweaks, like these, will go a long ways towards creating a more relaxed you!

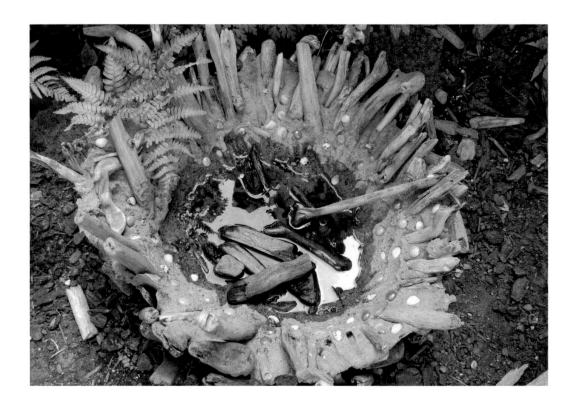

"A wise man adapts himself to circumstances as water shapes itself
to the vessel that contains it."   ~ Chinese Proverb

Adapt to Changing Circumstances

Mary became increasingly frail and susceptible to falls the last year. Wanting his mom to be able to stay in her own home, her son, Derek, built a sturdy wooden ramp so she wouldn't have to climb steps to the door. He also hired part-time caregivers and stopped by once a day. This arrangement seemed perfect until two weeks ago when an ambulance was called to her home. Because of a fall, Mary was transferred to the nearest ER, and then to the home of Derek and his wife who are providing care, at least for now.

Adjustments have been ongoing, both for Mary and her family, but such is the nature of caregiving! Just when we think we have things figured out, and a situation stabilized, it shifts again. How frustrating this can be, particularly if we are averse to change! Caregivers do well, then, to foster a flexible attitude, because change will be a constant.

Flexibility implies a willingness to adapt to changing circumstances and to shift priorities accordingly. It means letting go of strongly held opinions about how things should be done, and instead, being open to new approaches, sometimes suggested by the person for whom we are caring. What's more, flexibility requires less effort than trying to predict, plan for, or prevent the changes over which we have little or no control.

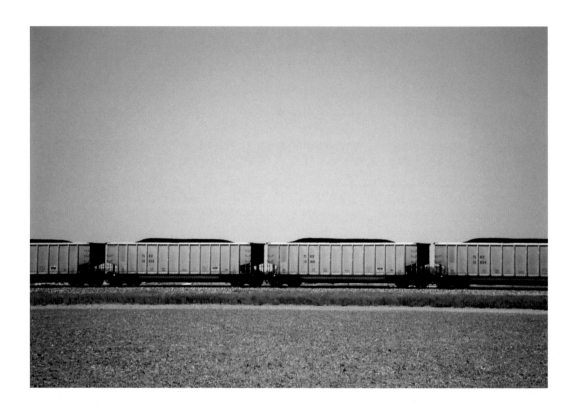

"It's not easy taking my problems one at a time when they refuse to get in line."   ~ Ashleigh Brilliant

Learn to Compartmentalize

Leaving the hospital after visiting a friend, I spotted the nurse who had just been in my friend's room talking on her cellphone. Her tone of voice demonstrated a high level of stress and agitation. How could she possibly go back inside and focus on patient care?

Personal problems had followed this nurse to work, just as they do for many us, and they impact our ability to provide quality and safe care. But, separating the world of work from our personal lives can seem next to impossible, unless we've learned how to compartmentalize. Compartmentalizing is the ability to focus on one aspect or "compartment" of our lives at a time. It's not unlike the storage containers on my garage shelves with holiday decorations in one, memorabilia in another, and old dishes in yet another. Keeping like things together, I feel more organized and efficient.

 Imagine a "container" or "compartment" for storing personal problems while providing care to another. Setting personal agendas aside allows you to give full attention to the tasks of the moment, and, it promotes a safer, calmer, more efficient you. Later, away from work, take the issues needing attention out of safekeeping, and try to address them. Leaving problems compartmentalized indefinitely is likely to create a whole other set of problems!

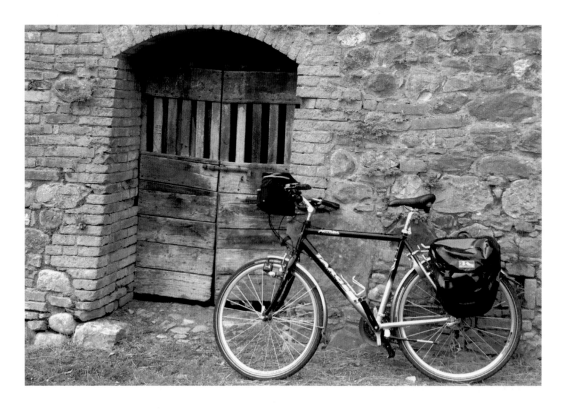

"We do not stop exercising because we grow old;
we grow old because we stop exercising."
~ Dr. Kenneth Cooper M.D.

Exercise

After drinking my cup of coffee this morning, I reasoned the weather too hot to go for a walk. I'll go to the gym later, after a scheduled lunch date with my granddaughter, I decided. But, after spending a delightful hour with her, there were other excuses: too tired, too much to do, too sweltering to ride my bike to the gym.

Finding the time and motivation to exercise is a challenge, and I can easily rationalize my way out of it. Caregivers, in particular, have legitimate sounding excuses: "I'm pooped!" or "I have too many other things on my plate." However, day after day of neglecting a walk, jog, bicycle ride, or gym time is counterproductive to caregiving. Exercise, after all, creates stamina, allowing us to work, play, and sleep at consistently higher levels. As one nurse put it, "If we tended to our bodies the way we care for others, we'd be a lot healthier, and we'd set a better example!"

A few simple tactics help me maintain an exercise routine: imagining the sense of accomplishment I'll feel afterwards; viewing my exercise as a part-time job—"showing up" is what I do; alternating my mode of exercise; adding a class to my repertoire; inviting a friend to go with me sometimes; and reminding myself that a little is better than nothing when time is short. What tactics will motivate you to get moving this day?

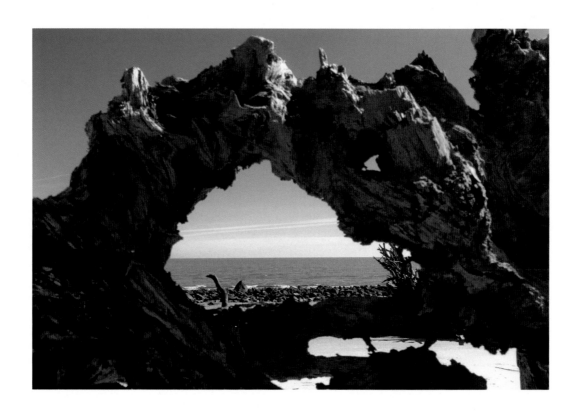

"The last of the human freedoms is to choose one's attitude in any given set of circumstance."   ~ Victor Frankl

Monitor Your Attitude

A very long box, with a new pair of cross-country skis inside, was delivered to my doorstep. A thank-you letter from the outdoor gear company was enclosed, and on the back side of the letter, the company's motto titled "Attitude." While I've seen similar versions before, I liked theirs, and wish to share an edited portion of it with you.

"... Attitude is one of the few things in life in which we have a true choice. We cannot change what is fated to happen [including the events in our lives and the actions of other people]. What we can change, however, is our reaction to such things with the attitude we adopt. Attitude is a choice we make every minute of every day. It is a state of mind that no one can take from us. If we are in control of our attitudes, we are in command of our lives. And that is the best way to live."

As caregivers, we tend to the needs of those who often have a myriad of challenges. Simultaneously, we might be struggling with our own problems. Telling someone to "keep your chin up" is not usually helpful, but modeling a positive mindset is more likely to have an impact. We do this by focusing on the things that are going well, on the blessings of each day, and on the areas of our lives where we do have control. In what ways are you modeling a positive attitude this day?

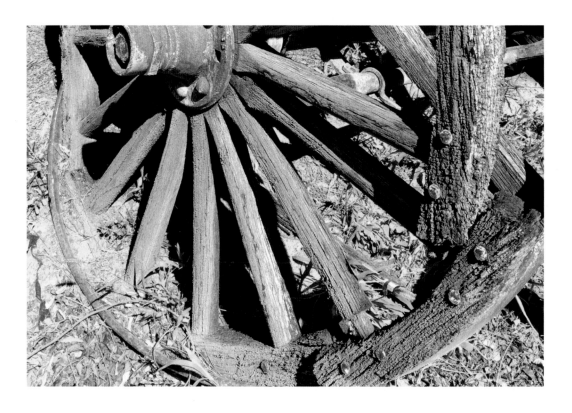

"A person without a sense of humor is like a wagon without springs.
It's jolted by every pebble on the road."

~ Henry Ward Beecher

Laugh Often

Not long ago, at our favorite coffee house, three dear friends and I deliberated the not-so-fun aspects of growing older. What started out as a depressing conversation morphed into hysterical laughter as we described the less-than-flattering parts of our bodies where the aging process has already taken a toll. I left our conversation feeling relaxed, lighter, and with a sense of commonality and camaraderie.

Yes, laughter has many benefits! It relaxes muscles, decreases pain, and boosts the immune system. Lessened anxiety and reduced stress are other pluses. Perhaps best of all, laughter facilitates the bonding of relationships, enhancing our ability to work and play together. Even an occasional laugh with the one(s) for whom we're giving care can reduce tension and encourage cooperation.

Telling ourselves to laugh more is not good enough, however. Rather, we need to set aside time with friends or colleagues for enjoyment and laughter—occasions to share funny stories, personal blunders, and goofy interactions. A mutually established ground rule could be that topics pertaining to caregiving duties and workplace politics be off limits. While these issues need to be addressed in their own time and manner, protecting social gatherings for more pleasurable interactions is critical!

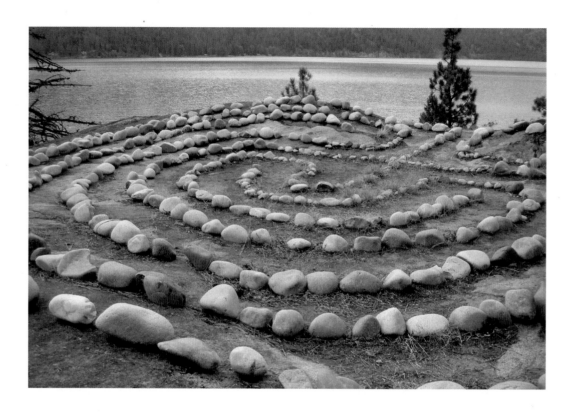

"Trust in the Lord with all your heart and lean not on your own understanding; in all your ways acknowledge Him, and He will direct your paths."   ~ Proverbs 3:5

Lean Not on Your Own Understanding

My husband traveled 800 miles to be with his dying mother. His sisters had told him it was time to come home if he wished to see her alive. He arrived with the intent of being present when his mom died, but, after a week, his mom looked no closer to death than when he arrived. One day, the hospice nurse told him, in private: "You might consider saying goodbye to your mom now, and going on home. She could be hanging on because she's afraid of hurting you." My spouse listened, said his goodbyes, and left for home. Less than ten hours later he was notified that his mother had passed.

A degree of mystery always accompanies our care for another. For example, it's tough, if not impossible, to understand the timing of a death, and the rationale—if there is any—for pain and suffering. We may question why it's him or her and not me who is ill or incapacitated, or the reasons why some die so young. Fortunately, the repetitive "why" questions surrounding a situation eventually fade to the background as our energies shift to finding the way forward and making the necessary adjustments. The good news from the writer of Proverbs is that we have a trusted guide on the journey—wherever it may lead. This too is a great mystery, as well as a remarkable gift!

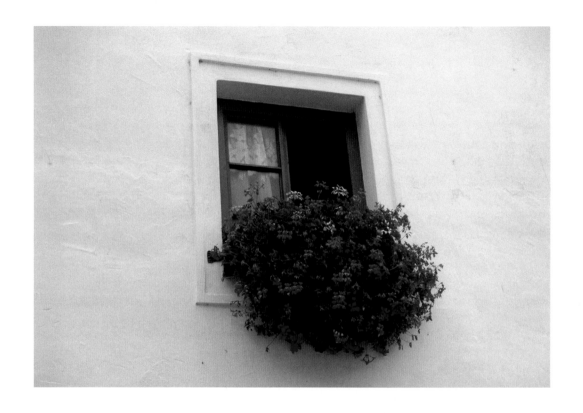

"Love begins by taking care of the closest ones—
the ones at home."   ~ Mother Teresa

Nurture Your Close Relationships

My friend, Lila, works a 9 to 5 job. Then, she heads to the home of her elderly parents to fix dinner and perform needed household tasks. She considers her daily visits vital to their well-being. Ask Lila how things are at home and she acknowledges her family is feeling slighted, and that time with friends has become a rarity.

Having time and energy for friends and family is difficult when we're busy helping those with seemingly greater needs! However, we risk having vital sources of support and camaraderie wither and die if we don't give them our attention too. Marriages, in particular, suffer if partners don't make time to nurture each other or the relationship.

Think about the persons with whom you feel closest. Then, conduct a self-audit using the questions below to determine if you're holding up your end of those relationships. If you see areas for needed improvement, commit to making one or two small changes.

~ Do I call to check in or initiate time to get together?
~ Do I ask what's going on in their lives and take a genuine interest?
~ Do I regularly express appreciation for the ways they show support?

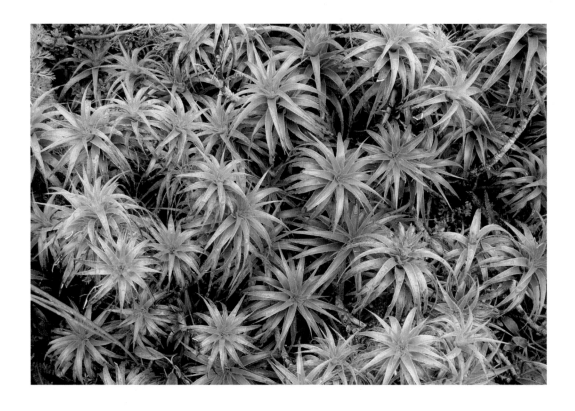

"Authenticity is the alignment of head, mouth, heart, and feet —
thinking, saying, feeling, and doing the same thing — consistently."
~ Lance Secretan

Live with Authenticity

Did your ever catch your parents doing something they had instructed you not to do? And when you pointed it out, they might have responded, "Do as I say; not as I do!" This is an example of how we are taught to live inauthentic lives. When we live authentic lives, however, we do just the opposite—our actions reflect our words; we do what we say we'll do. Two synonyms for authenticity are genuineness and truthfulness—attributes that make us trustworthy, dependable, and consistent caregivers.

One sure way to monitor your authenticity level is to ask others for periodic feedback, using the following questions for starters: (Be sure to answer these for yourself first so you will know if your self-assessment is accurate!)

~ Am I a dependable and trustworthy caregiver and/or health care team member?
~ Do my actions line up with my words? In other words, do I walk the talk?
~ Am I respectful of the rights, opinions, and differences of others?

While the quest for authenticity is a journey, not a destination, an honest appraisal of ourselves, and meaningful feedback from others, can help us keep our feet on the path.

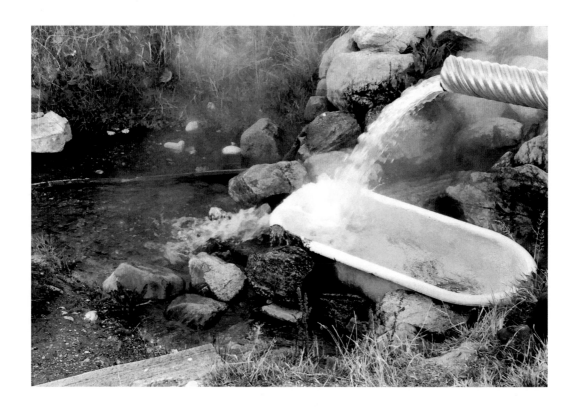

"Thousands have lived without love, not one without water."
~ W.H. Auden

Stay Hydrated

Two mugs of coffee to wake me up, a mid-afternoon cup of tea, and a full glass of water to swallow my vitamins is hardly enough to keep my body working at an optimum level. On good days, I remember to drink more. Other days, I forget.

Water makes up about 60% of our body weight, and every one of our internal systems depends on it. Water flushes out toxins, gets nutrients to cells, and keeps tissues moist. It can also help curb our appetite, an aid in controlling weight. However, since water is lost through the breath, urine, and skin, we have to replenish it or we're apt to feel fatigued and sluggish—not conducive to a caregiver's optimal performance.

Often-heard advice is to drink eight 8-ounce glasses of fluid, primarily water, each day. However, the eight-glasses-a-day rule needs to be modified depending on our activity level, health status, and the environment we're in.

A good measure of hydration is, of course, our level of thirst. But, since thirst is easy to ignore, a more reliable indicator is urine color: clear or light yellow means we're probably okay. Dark yellow urine means it's time to fill up a large glass or water bottle and start sipping away!

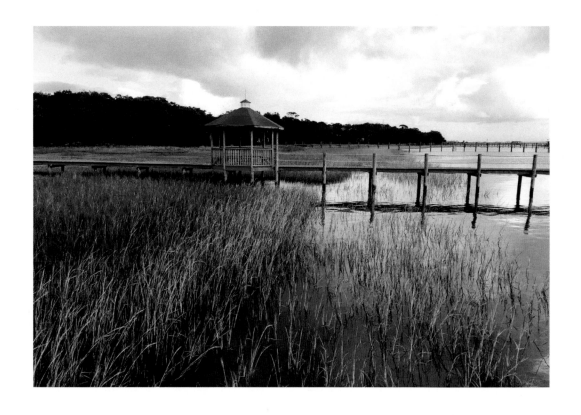

"As you walk and eat and travel, be where you are.
Otherwise you will miss most of your life."   ~ Buddha

Be Where You Are

Watching my grandson savor grandma's made-to-order deluxe ice cream sundae when he comes to visit, delights me. His smile reveals sheer pleasure as he examines the tantalizing presentation and experiences the smooth and cool, sweet and salty sensations in his mouth. Unbeknownst to Luke, he is embodying mindfulness.

Mindfulness is paying careful attention to the present moment, including sights, sounds, tastes, smells, and even bodily sensations. Being mindful—whether I'm walking, eating, driving, chopping vegetables, or caring for others—prevents runaway thoughts of the past and worries about the future. But, staying in the moment takes a lot of effort as my thoughts have had a lifetime of free rein!

I offer this mindfulness exercise to practice throughout the day: With eyes open or closed, take a moment to focus attention only on your breathing, trying not to change or modify it. When your mind wanders—and it always does—gently, without self-judgment, return attention to your breathing. If you are experiencing sadness, grief, anger, or another difficult emotion, gently bring it to your attention, and notice where you are carrying the feeling in your body. Then, place your hand on that part of your body in a spirit of compassion. Do this for a minute or two and see what happens.

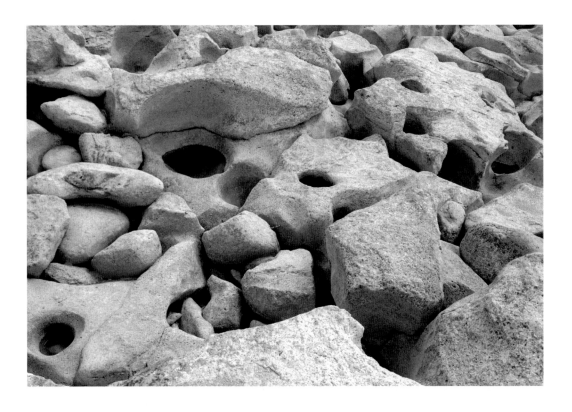

"We burn out, not because we don't care, but because we don't grieve
. . .because we have allowed our hearts to become so filled with loss
that we have no room left to care."   ~ Rachel Remen, MD

Grieve the Losses

My endearing eighty-year old client died unexpectedly. I had seen him a week before, yet only learned of his death in the newspaper. When my initial shock had worn off, I felt sad that I didn't have a chance to say good-bye.

Yes, we caregivers grieve—whether the death is of a loved one or a patient! We grieve, too, as we watch someone decline, anticipating their death. Because grief is painful and difficult, however, we often try to minimize or ignore it, which may work in the short term, but not over the long haul. I've seen many a caregiver seemingly breeze through death after death. But, I've also witnessed the cost when grief stays bottled-up: chronic pain, work absenteeism, overeating, alcohol or drug abuse, and non-stop busyness.

So how do we confront grief without letting it overwhelm us? After learning of the death of my elderly client, I called a trusted colleague—a good listener—to share my sorrow. I read and reread the obituary, reviewed my case notes, and considered what I had learned from my work with him. In other times of loss, I've attended memorial services, visited the gravesite, lit a candle in his or her name, and sought counseling. And, I've filled scores of pages in my journals when I was unable to express my grief verbally. Think back over the losses you've had, and the various ways you processed your grief.

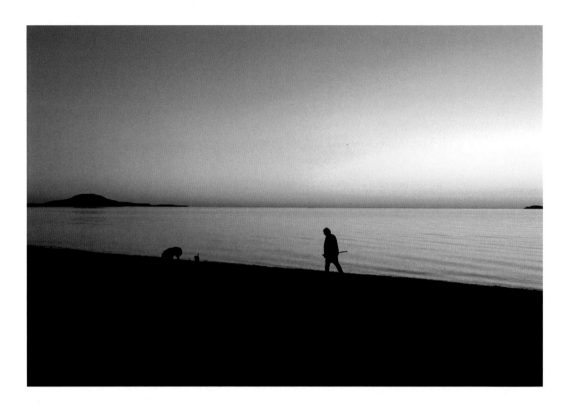

"The best remedy for those who are afraid, lonely or unhappy is to go outside, somewhere where they can be quiet, alone with the heavens, nature and God."   ~ Anne Frank

Take Your N Vitamin

A variety of studies demonstrate that regular exposure to nature positively impacts the way we function. For instance, hospital patients exposed to tree views tend to need fewer pain medications and get released from the hospital sooner. Likewise, spending time in nature has been found to benefit people who are depressed, anxious, and angry. Richard Louv, author of *Last Child in the Woods*, refers to nature as the "N Vitamin." He writes, "Humans are hard-wired to love and need exposure to the natural world," and "the more high-tech our lives become, the more nature we need."

While I sometimes drive to the mountains or head to the foothills near my home for a nature fix, more often I get exposure to the natural world by walking in the neighborhood, tending my garden box, or watching squirrels run up and down the fence line. To heighten awareness of my surroundings, I often take a camera outside. Then, I'm likely to notice the bed of orange poppies next to a battered fence, the reflection of cumulus clouds in a street puddle, a black cat chasing a robin from his perch, and the unusual papery bark on a river birch tree.

Have you been taking your N vitamin? If not, start today—if even for a few minutes. You'll be a happier, healthier caregiver as a result.

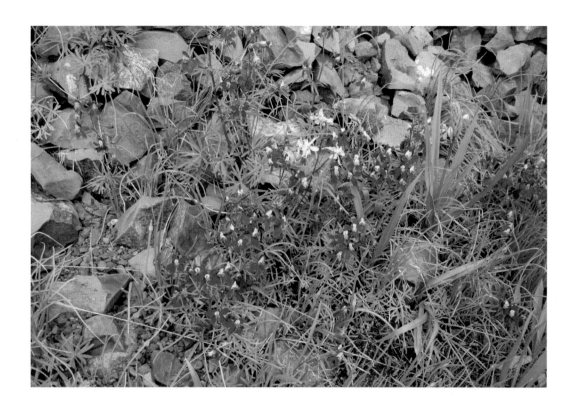

"Kindness is in our power, even when fondness is not."

~ Samuel Johnson

Respond Creatively to Mistreatment

A group of Starbucks employees collected groceries for a man who had blatantly robbed the contents of their tip jar. While many folks suggested filing charges, the workers chose to respond with love and compassion rather than revenge. They did the unexpected and creatively turned a negative incident into something positive.

This too was the spirit of the late Nelson Mandela. He lived through years of imprisonment and endured torture from his captors, but he chose to forgive those who hurt him; he responded in improbable ways that garnered respect and inspired hope.

Sometimes the people we care for say hurtful things or behave in cruel ways. Not knowing an appropriate response, we tend to absorb the negative energy that comes our way. A build-up of tension from these incidents makes us vulnerable to burnout and self-destructive behaviors. The next time you encounter undesirable behavior, take a deep breath and consider your alternatives. You do have choices in how to respond! For instance, you could say something like this: "Your comment or action was hurtful to me." Or, depending on the situation, you might decide to overlook the negative words or actions and respond with kindness. Then again, you might want to consult with someone you trust before you respond.

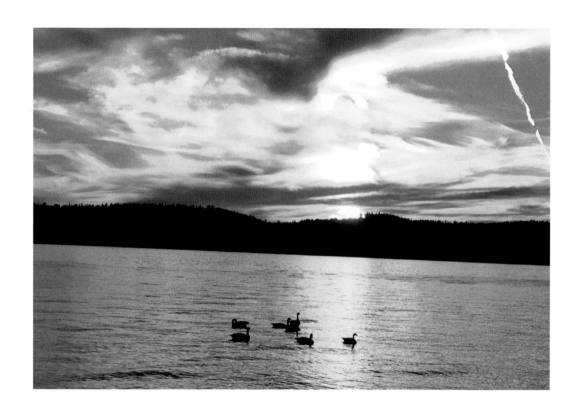

"Adopt the pace of nature, her secret is patience."
~ Ralph Waldo Emerson

Slow Down, Be Present

My 96-year-old mother lives in an assisted-living facility, and because she resides in a neighboring state, I'm able to visit her often. Upon entering mom's world, I'm reminded again of how slow her life has become—from shuffling with a walker down the hallway to methodically taking off her shoes at bedtime. She's unhurried in accepting my suggestions as well. "We'll see," or "Let me think about it" are common responses. Of course, I want to fix any problems I see right away.

Jane Gross, in her 2012 memoir, *Bittersweet Season: Caring for Our Aging Parents and Ourselves*, writes about the need to slow down when caring for another: "I sprinted when I should have cautiously watched my step. . .barked orders when I should have discussed things with my mother. You can't bulldoze your way through this [caregiving] like a work project." She goes on to say, "Some things are in your hands and some are not. What is vital and well within your control is being present in a consoling way. . ."

Gross' words encourage me to slow down, stay present, and offer support rather than spring into fix-it mode. This is not easy for a take-charge caregiver like me, but I do feel a sense of freedom in knowing I don't have to make it all okay.

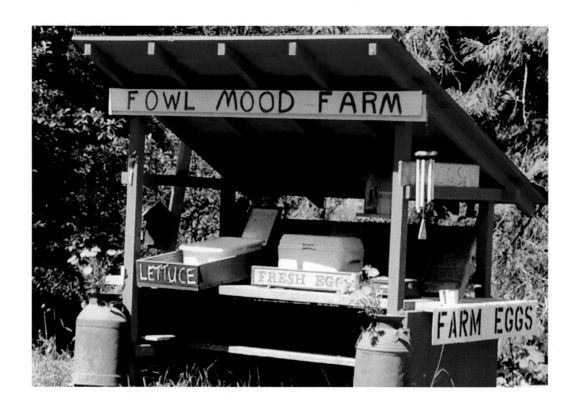

"Without enough sleep, we all become tall two-year-olds."
~ JoJo Jensen

Get Your Sleep

In an episode of PBS's British comedy, *Doc Martin*, Martin's ditzy secretary keeps falling asleep at her computer because of sleep deprivation. The culprit? Her brother's loud snoring! One night, out of sheer exhaustion, she gets up and puts a pillow over his face, acting out (humorously) her desire to suffocate him!

Lack of sleep, night after night, can indeed cause us to act in foolish ways, and it robs us of patience, energy, efficiency and the ability to solve problems. Yet sleep deprivation is acknowledged as a problem by every family caregiver I know, and it's an all too common reality for professional caregivers as well—particularly for those who "take call" at night or work varying shifts.

What to do? First, acknowledge how lack of sleep is impacting your life. Then, try a few simple tips known to improve sleep. For example, stay consistent in the times you go to bed and get up; create calming bedtime rituals like a warm bath or a cup of herbal tea; avoid caffeine and alcohol late in the day; get out of bed and engage in a quiet activity if you can't fall asleep within thirty minutes; and find someone to regularly spell you if lack of sleep is due to caregiving demands during the night. Finally, consult with your doctor if nothing else works.

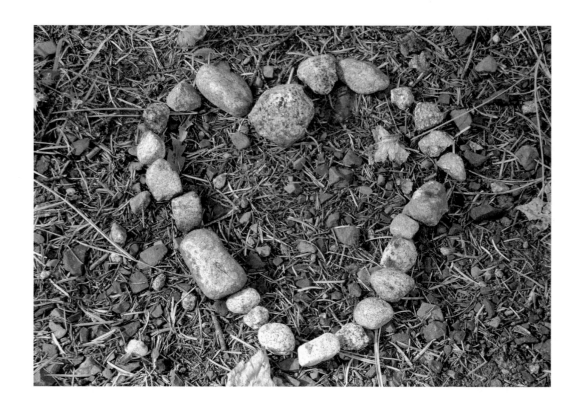

"I want to write, but more than that I want to bring out all kinds of things that lie buried in my heart."   ~ Anne Frank

Keep a Journal

A box of old journals sits in my basement closet. On the box flaps I've scrawled in bold letters, "If I die, please shred or burn these." That's because I don't censor what I write. My journals have and will continue to be safe outlets for my anger, sadness, grief, worry, and joy. These emotions, and others, I express with words, scribbles, and drawings, paying no heed to grammar, spelling, or being nice.

I believe caregivers of all kinds could benefit from a regular journal writing practice. It's a form of self-care that releases pent-up emotions, clears the mind, lowers stress, and boosts the immune system. The following tips can help you get started:

~ Use any type of notebook with blank or lined pages, and a favorite pen or pencil.
~ Write 5-10 minutes a day, and/or whenever you feel the urge.
~ Write about anything on your heart and mind as this writing is only for you.
~ Describe your feelings in detail: "I feel tense like a knotted up rope." or "I feel anxious like dark clouds gathering before a storm."
~ Depict a feeling with crayons or paint when words don't come.
~ Try writing some of your journal entries, in the form of a letter you don't send, to God, a person who mistreated you, or the one you're caring for.

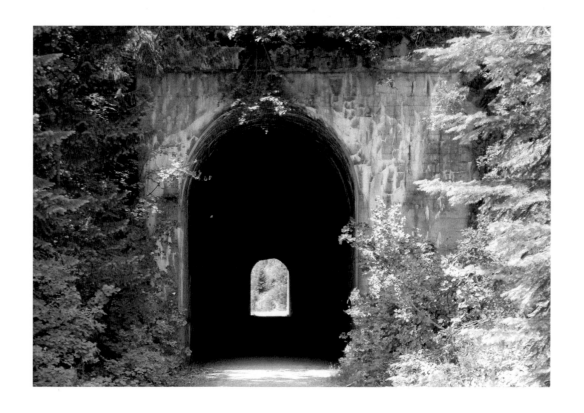

"Forgiveness isn't something we do for others;
we do it so we can get well and move on."   ~ Anonymous

Choose to Forgive

"My dad was never there for me as a child, and now I'm supposed to take care of him!" "My mom is disrespectful and rude, yet I continue to care for her out of guilt!" "My coworker never lifts a finger to help, and I'm angry!" "Some days I am hurried and harried as I give care; then later I get down on myself!"

These feelings of animosity and resentment are all too common, adding to the day-to-day burden of caregiving. They keep us chained to injuries of the recent or long-ago past, and rob us of energy and pleasure. Forgiving others and ourselves is the key to releasing those chains. But, let me be clear, forgiving is not forgetting, or making excuses for someone's behavior. Neither does forgiving demand an apology or assume a restored relationship. Rather, it is choosing not to punish or get even with the one who wronged us. It is making a conscious choice to focus on the here and now rather than on grievances of yesterday or yesteryear!

Bringing to mind the flawed past of the person who caused our hurt helps us forgive, as does seeking the guidance of a counselor or spiritual mentor when we feel stuck, unable to heal. Writing "I forgive you for. . ." can be beneficial as well. Even though I may not feel ready to forgive, repeating those words reminds me of my intent.

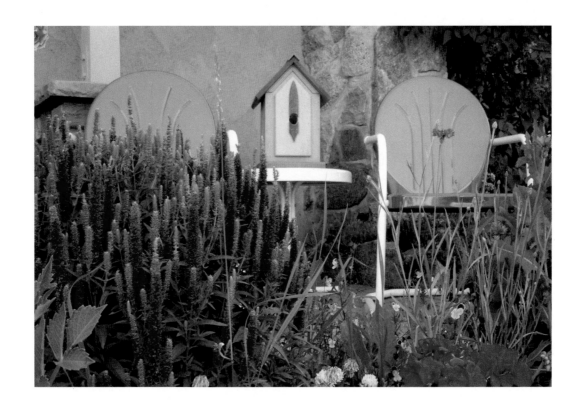

"Life is lived in the pauses, not the events."   ~ Hugh Prather

Make Time for Leisure

Busyness, like cleanliness, is next to godliness, or at least that was my childhood take-away message. But, I also learned that one day each week—the Sabbath—was set aside for morning church services, followed by an afternoon of rest and leisure. Extended naps, reading, and relaxed drives in the country were the norm.

Though I frequently attend worship services on Sunday, I seldom set aside the rest of the day for sheer leisure. My distractions are numerous: The computer allows me to work from home—as I'm doing right now. My cell phone—usually at my side—lures me into responding to texts and emails, and a stack of mail beckons me to the office.

Thankfully, I'm not quite as driven as I used to be. I've learned that it's impossible to be effective and efficient in my labors, particularly in my helping roles, without making time for rest and relaxation. Therefore, I try to regularly incorporate activities like hiking, bicycling, reading for pleasure, playing the ukulele, and socializing with friends into my life. Leisure time brings renewed perspective, balance, and fresh energy for my work, and I assume it does for you as well. When do you make time for leisure, and what activities bring needed renewal?

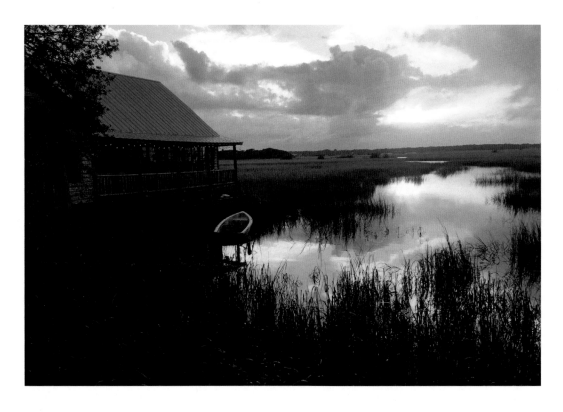

"Man's words and actions presume always a crisis near at hand, but she [nature] is forever silent and unpretending."
~ Henry David Thoreau

Practice Equanimity

A stay-at-home mom with two toddlers told me she was practicing "equanimity," an assignment given by her yoga instructor. This meant striving for calmness, composure, and an even temper, especially in high stress situations.

Equanimity is a terrific practice for caregivers of all kinds, not just young mothers! After all, stressful situations arise and those in our charge get upset and angry. However, when we manage to keep a cool and unflustered demeanor, even while churning on the inside, the other is more likely to calm down.

Taking some deep breaths helps us stay composed. Keeping in mind that the other's upset is not necessarily about us, but about their situation or lack of skills in managing difficult emotions, helps too. Finally, responding with empathy, not judgment, has a calming effect on them and us—"I hear how upset you are. Tell me what's going on."

A quiet lily pond in an area I sometimes walk represents the equanimity I desire in challenging situations. A busy community of plant and animal life thrives below the pond's surface, but few clues of that activity exist as I observe the glassy surface. Is there an image that represents the equanimity you strive for?

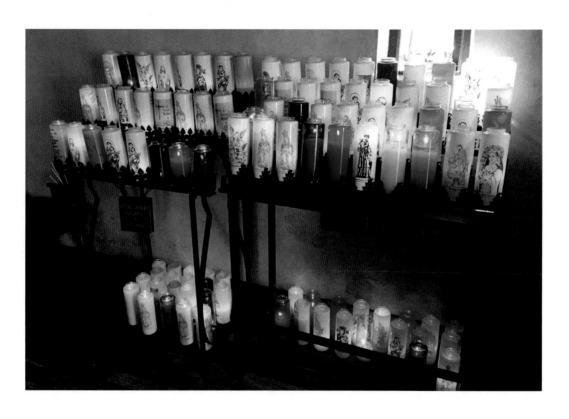

"In everyone's life, at some time, our inner fire goes out. . .We
should all be thankful for those people who rekindle
the inner spirit."   ~ Albert Schweitzer

Seek Support

Peggy stopped meeting me for walks after her husband became homebound following a stroke. Concerned that he could fall, Peggy stayed close to home. Consequently, her social connections began fading away, and feelings of isolation and loneliness ensued.

A 39-year-old mother of three died at home soon after I arrived for a hospice nurse visit. Her age and young children touched me greatly, and I needed to talk about it with my colleagues. But, upon returning to the office, I discovered that most were gone for the day. I felt alone and unsupported!

While both of the above scenarios are very different, the commonality seems to be a yearning for connectedness and support in the midst of caregiving. Without these ingredients, self-confidence dwindles, discouragement surfaces, and the potential for burnout increases. If you're a family caregiver, arrange for a "sitter" so you can get away to spend time with friends. Also, consider joining a caregiver support group where there are others "in the same boat" as you are in. Professional caregivers: discuss with your supervisor the possibility of regular peer support group sessions. Ideally led by a trained facilitator, peer support groups can reduce the emotional stress of caregiving, encourage self-care measures, and serve to "rekindle the inner spirit."

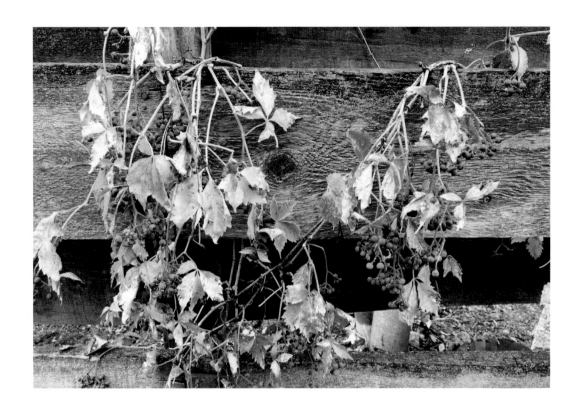

"Letting go means accepting what is, exactly as it is, without fear, resistance, or a struggle for control."   ~ Iyanla Vanzant

Let Go

Jon is nauseated and sluggish for several days after his chemotherapy. He arrives home from his treatments wanting to sleep and be left alone. Since he lives by himself, with no family nearby, I call to check in: "What sounds good to eat?" What can I bring you?" "Nothing," is the usual response, even when I suggest his favorite flavor of milkshake. I feel helpless and concerned, wanting somehow to lessen his distress.

Jon knows that his friends and I want to help in every way possible. However, when we provide food without first asking, or do other kind favors without checking with him, he's quick to point out, with his sometimes lack of diplomacy, that we're doing it more for ourselves than we are for him. He claims he'll let us know when he needs our help. For now, he can manage just fine.

A lesson that I am relearning for the umpteenth time is that sometimes the best way to help is to accept the fact that I cannot help. In Jon's situation, for instance, I'm a listener and supporter, not a helper. I check in by phone on a consistent basis, and I try to listen really carefully when Jon needs to vent. Sometimes I sneak in a piece of advice, but back off quickly when he comes back with a rebuttal. Not helping is more difficult than I ever imagined!

"In the end, only three things matter:

How well we have lived.
How well we have loved.
How well we have learned to let go."

~Jack Kornfield

Index by Topic

Physical Health:

       Breathe Slowly-17

       Consider Self-Care a Part-Time Job-3

       Eat Wisely-31

       Exercise-45

       Get Your Sleep-69

       Stay Hydrated-57

Mental Fitness:

       Be Where You Are-59

       Cultivate Gratitude-5

       Keep Perspective-19

       Maintain Hope-33

       Monitor Your Attitude-47

Emotional Release:

       Count to 10 When Triggered-21

       Grieve the Losses-61

       Keep a Journal-71

       Laugh Often-49

       Own Your Feelings-7

       Seek Outlets for Difficult Emotions-35

       Practice Equanimity-77

Spiritual Connectedness:
      Acknowledge the Sacred-9
      Choose to Forgive-73
      Discover the Power of Two Questions-37
      Lean Not on Your Own Understanding-51
      Live with Authenticity-55
      Memorize a Prayer or Mantra-23
      Take Your N Vitamin-63
Friend, Family & Leisure Time:
      Ask for Help-11
      Eliminate the Non-Essentials-39
      Leave Your Shoes at the Door-25
      Make Time for Leisure-75
      Nurture Your Close Relationships-53
      Seek Support-79
      Strive for Balance-15
Caregiver Strategies:
      Accept Your Vulnerabilities-13
      Adapt to Changing Circumstances-41
      Respond Creatively to Mistreatment-65
      Establish Boundaries-29
      Learn to Compartmentalize-43
      Let Go-81
      Recognize Your Limits-27
      Slow Down, Be Present-67

Other Books by This Author

The Nature of Grief: Photographs and Words for Reflection and Healing
(Resources for Grief, 2009, 2015)

When Shiner Died: A Children's Book About Pet Loss
(Resources for Grief, 2010)

Grief Support Mailings: User Manual and CD
(Resources for Grief, 2010)

Eight-Session Grief Support Group Leader's Manual
(Resources for Grief, 2013)

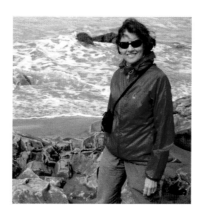

About the Author: Rebecca S. Hauder, a Registered Nurse, Licensed Clinical Professional Counselor, and Marriage and Family Therapist, worked twelve years in the hospice setting. There she witnessed and experienced firsthand the rewards and struggles of providing care to the elderly, sick, and dying. Since her years working in hospice, Rebecca has provided counseling to professional and family caregivers, and to those experiencing major life transitions, including loss and grief. She has created bereavement resources for individuals, hospice organizations, and funeral homes, and writes a "Self-Care Tip of the Month" for family and professional caregivers (www. resourcesforgrief.com/resources). Rebecca also serves as an adjunct professor for Boise State University's Department of Counselor Education. Currently residing in Boise, Idaho, she is married with two grown children and four grandchildren.

List of Author's Photographs:

Cover: Ponderosa State Park, McCall, Idaho
Page 2:   Moeraki Boulders, Oamaru, New Zealand
Page 4:   Foothills, Boise, Idaho
Page 6:   Hull's Gulch, Boise, Idaho
Page 8:   Palm Desert, California
Page 10: Maui, Hawaii (Photo: Leah VanVactor)
Page 12: McCall, Idaho
Page 14: Kekerengu, New Zealand
Page 16: Wyoming countryside
Page 18: Boise, Idaho
Page 20: LaPine, Oregon
Page 22: McCall, Idaho
Page 24: A winery in Washington State
Page 26: Paradise Point Camp, McCall, Idaho
Page 28: Arches National Park, Utah
Page 30: Pike Street Market, Seattle, Washington
Page 32: Payette National Forest, near Burgdorf, Idaho
Page 34: Payette Lake, McCall, Idaho
Page 36: Arches National Park, Utah
Page 38: Charlie's Garden, McCall, Idaho
Page 40: Kekerengu, New Zealand

Page 42: Plains of Colorado
Page 44: Umbria region, Italy
Page 46: Jekyll Island, South Carolina
Page 48: Farewell Bend State Park, Oregon
Page 50: Paradise Point Camp, McCall, Idaho
Page 52: A village in Austria
Page 54: A garden in New Zealand
Page 56: Burgdorf, Idaho
Page 58: Mantanzas Marsh, St. Augustine, Florida
Page 60: Snake River, Caldron Linn, Murtaugh, Idaho
Page 62: Loreto beach, Baja Sur, Mexico
Page 64: Ponderosa State Park, McCall, Idaho
Page 66: Payette Lake, McCall, Idaho
Page 68: Salt Spring Island, BC, Canada
Page 70: Ponderosa State Park, McCall, Idaho
Page 72: Hiawatha Rail Trail, near Wallace, Idaho
Page 74: Artizen Gallery, McCall, Idaho
Page 76: Anastasia Island, Florida
Page 78: Cathedral Basilica of St. Augustine, Florida
Page 80: Hill Road, Boise, Idaho

Made in the USA
Columbia, SC
26 March 2020